As The Chair Turns...

Tips & Snips of Advice for Your Journey Behind the Chair

Dedicated to the past, the present, and the future professionals.

Acknowledgements

I never dreamed that writing a book for hairdressers could be this much fun!

To Cindy McGuire…Your belief in me and my hair-brained ideas over the years has been unceasing. This book could not have been completed without your valuable time, insights, and creative perspectives. I appreciate and respect your input and expertise in the fine detail you enthusiastically dedicated to this book. Having you as my sounding board has brought to life the publication of *As The Chair Turns…* A very heartfelt "Thank You" for your outstanding presence in my life and for making the process fun!

To my mother, Jackie Baker…All my life I watched you with admiration, for you had the gift of making people feel special when they were around you. Your little but mighty salon held special memories for everyone who entered and your love for people out-shined the stars. Many of the words and much of the abundant spirit of this book belongs to you, my dear mother, for you made a lasting impression on me that created a love and passion for my work as a hairdresser. You empowered me to want to share this amazing professional spirit with all of my fellow beauty professionals. I love you, Ma.

To my "POPS", my DADDY!...I can't tell you enough how much your love and support has given to my family and me. Of all the people in my life you have been my rock, my life mentor, my father, my daddy, my trusted friend. Your strength and encouragement have given me all the tools to survive, values to live by and memories I will cherish. Having you by my side made my life much simpler - you were always THERE, always ready to help me. Words can't describe what that did for my self-esteem. Just knowing that I could count on you made me who I am today!! I'm a blessed woman to have such a wonderful father to guide and love me in everything that I do. I love you, Daddy!

To Gramma Donna...Thank you forever, for being the awesome woman that you are! You were my very first client who believed in my abilities and had an open mind that has allowed me to explore all aspects of this business. You were the one person who never said no and let me make mistakes with on your precious head. Your love and devotion to our family is so beautiful. You give us the morals and "proper rules" to live by. I value everything that you do and all of the heartwarming memories that you create. There is only one Gramma Donna, in my life.

Kari-Jo…My biggest Cheerleader! My sister, my best friend! A big "thank you" for everything!! There is nothing you wouldn't do for me and I know that. Having you by my side has injected my enthusiasm for anything I ever wanted to accomplish. Words are not enough for you, my dear sister. My heart is swollen with happiness for the friendship that we have and the bond that will never be broken.

To my husband, Marty…my lifelong partner. Your love for me has allowed many opportunities to grow and become fully human. I am tremendously grateful for your honesty and constructive criticism that pushes me to go a little further in any task that I encounter. Sharing my life with you is the most powerful, positive energy force that I have in my life and everything I do is a deep reflection of you.

To my girls, Camille and Marie…My deepest thanks to you both for understanding what I wanted to accomplish. Your continual support and zealous attitudes have nurtured the dreams to become real. Thank you for putting up with all of my client traffic, and for believing in your mother's crazy world in the beauty business. My deepest wish is for you to find the same passion in your chosen career. xoxo.

Preface

Being a hairdresser is filled with the opportunity to explore expressions of yourself in a unique and challenging way. Inspiration is all around us, if we are open to the discovery within our environment. During the past twenty-five years in this business, I have been inspired to try many concepts; some worked, and some didn't. But the one thing that I learned is this is one fascinating business!

Your profession gives you the opportunity to continuously uncover yourself both professionally and personally. Your work is art, but the truth is, art is life. Creating works of art goes beyond the technical skills for today's hairdresser. This book gives insight to some of the truths about your career as well as powerful business skills that can lead to financial independence.

Whether you are a big salon owner or employee, an independent contractor, a seasoned stylist or an excited beauty school student…within these pages you will find encouraging insights that will reveal real-life situations and ideas that will help you understand the nature of our business and inspire you to enjoy the ride. The passion for sharing this information and education has been the heart and soul of my journey behind the chair.

Kathy Jager

In order to succeed in this increasingly competitive, diverse, mad but marvelous business, today's stylist must be educated in all areas of life.

READ ON!

You can have everything in life you want if you just help enough people get what they want.
Zig Zigler

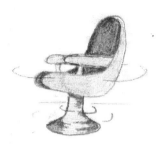

Stylin' And Smilin'

PROFESSIONAL PRIDE

When you think of the word "Professional", do you put it next to your name? Or is the status of the word too much for you to handle? Do you think you need a Ph.D. or BA after your name in order for you to receive the proper respect that comes with the word "professional"? Being a professional means that you take on added responsibility and that you are an achiever. It means that you place value in what you do and take pride in what and how you can offer your service to others. The word professional is a validation. It identifies you as a person with the right education, knowledge, skills, and talent.

If you choose to use the words "I am a professional" (and you should), you declare that you are one who is up to the challenges of the profession.

Position Yourself

Some people think that being a hairdresser is a flaky position, a mindless job you get when you lack education. Little do they know that this profession provides life-learning skills; skills that you need every day to manage well in this world. The technical aspect of our industry is important, but is secondary when it comes to providing customer service. People come to beauty professionals for their expertise and skill, but they also come for the human connection. They trust us to help them transform themselves inside and out. Clients place value on the human nature of our service - the part of our job to which very few other professions can relate. Our profession stands tall when you understand all that it takes to keep up with the daily demands of our jobs.

Gateway To Excellence

This industry has come a long way from the "beauty school dropouts" of the '50s when being a hairdresser was one of the only other options open to women besides being a homemaker or secretary. The industry has helped change the world for women, giving them education, powerful careers, impressive incomes, flexible hours, exciting work environments, and the best position to be able to make other people look and feel beautiful. Our industry has also opened the world's eyes to art, fashion, beauty, fitness, health, spirituality, business - the list is endless. The only limitation in this profession is our own.

People Power

We have the power to transform people's moods, the tools to beautify their souls and the creativity to make them look magnificent. The time you spend with your client can have an enormous impact on them, as most of the time they are coming for you to "fix" something in their life - not always their hair. Being a professional, you know that, so you put one of your many life-learning skills to work and dive in.

Enjoy Your Work

To be a beauty professional today means you wear many hats, all of which contribute to the most satisfying and gratifying profession available. Loving what you do daily makes your journey in the professional world exciting and fulfilling. It's often been said, "Love what you do you and you will never work a day in your life." So the next time someone asks you what you do for a living, tell him or her proudly, "I am a professional."

"Give the heavens above more than just a passing glance…"
Leeann Womack

Tips & Snips

List three reasons why you chose this profession:

Reason one:_____

Reason two:_____

Reason three:_____

NEW CLIENTS: THEY'RE EVERYWHERE!

There is nothing more discouraging to a hairdresser than to get out of beauty school, find the perfect salon to work in, have the excitement about all the great hair you're going to do, and then find yourself sitting, instead of standing behind the chair. It happens all the time. Why? Is it the salon owner's fault? The location? No! It's *your* business, and you have to take responsibility for it. You need to be *hungry*. You need to be *creative*. You need to be able to introduce yourself and build relationships with everyone you meet.

Grow Every Day

Every day you have potential clients. Think about it for a moment: you go to the same grocery store every week, the same bank, the same church, and the same kid's school. All of these places are great ways to meet new clientele. It is *up to you* to approach a new client with your business card in a comfortable way.

Your business depends on your participation.

Sure, salon owners market the salon for new clients, but the real way for you to get new clients is to be proactive as an *individual*. You have to constantly be building your clientele. This is a competitive business, and there are many reasons why people change salons. No matter how busy you are today, you can never become lax in acquiring and keeping your clientele.

Clients stay for a reason, a season or a lifetime. It is up to you to keep that client in your chair for a lifetime.

Ways To Build Your Business

✂   Begin with your existing clientele. Hold a promotion with your clients. One sure way is to have a sign that says, "Want a FREE haircut - ask me how!" Then tell them that for every client they send you, you'll give them a free haircut. Try it, it works!

✂   Go and pass out $5.00 off coupons or 50% off cards with your menu of services to every business that is in your neighborhood and introduce yourself personally.

✂   Network with your existing clients and their personal business. Host events together that would benefit both of you.

✂   Offer a gift certificate for ANY fund-raiser.

✂   Hold a drawing in your salon for clients to refer their friends and reward them with services.

These are just a few winning ideas to remind you that clients are everywhere. You just have to seek them out. REMEMBER: If it is to be, it is up to me!!!

"He who seeks rest finds boredom; he who seeks work finds rest."

Unknown

Tips & Snips

Name 3 places you will pass out your business cards today:

Place one:_____

Place two:_____

Place three:_____

MOVING ON

There is an old saying - *If you always do what you've always done, you'll always get what you've always gotten.* Now that might be great if you are content with your life, your finances, and your professional growth. But, what if being content just isn't enough? What about when the need to grow becomes so strong that it pushes you to challenge yourself to something new? Where do you go next? Do you change professions? Go back to school to get a new degree? Quit? Don't even think about it!

The day you graduated from your beauty college was the day a world of opportunities opened up for you. You just forgot, because you limited yourself to only one aspect of our profession. And I'm not saying that there is anything wrong with that - hairdressing is one of the best professions you could be in. But sometimes, even great hairdressers wonder what's next? The time to think about your next move is when the day-to-day working behind the chair just isn't as fulfilling as it once was. It is not that you don't enjoy your work, or the clients; it is about the challenge within yourself that creates the need for a change. This happens to a lot of hairdressers, especially seasoned pros.

But instead of looking outside of your profession, I suggest you sit down and evaluate your career with an open mind and remember that you have only tapped into one part of this dynamic industry. Being a beauty professional has many avenues for you to choose from and all you need is a friendly reminder of the other career opportunities that are available.

Think About Your Needs

Besides money, what is it that you need from your work that will challenge you and bring you daily happiness? Try to think about what you enjoy most about our field. Is it the artistry? The hands-on work, or do you prefer the connection with people? Knowing what it is that you like will help to take the guesswork out of your next move.

Step Out Of Your Box

Look into areas that interest you, but you were afraid to venture into. Perhaps you always admired platform artists but told yourself, "I could never do that."

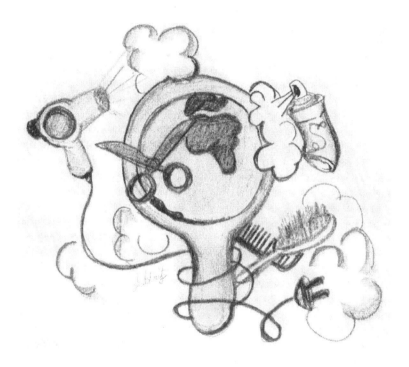

Or, perhaps you always wanted to be a fashion-model makeup artist, or a show event coordinator. All of these careers are open for you to try. You simply have to find what it is that interests you and *just do it.*

Make The Connection

Our industry is filled with the right people who will gladly HELP you to get to where you need to go. You must make the first move, and that is to start networking with people in your profession who are already doing what you want to do.

If you can't find anyone then begin your journey by going to classes and seminars on the subject or career that interests you. Your peers would love to hook you up with what they love to do; it is part of our industry's nature. When you're excited, they're excited to share with you.

Which Way Do You Go?

This is the hardest part - deciding a direction. The first thing to do is to review your choices. Of course, there are basic choices, such as stylist, colorist, nail tech, and esthetician. But there's a world of other choices as well. You might have forgotten that our profession offers endless opportunities. And there are ways for the experienced professional to expand his or her career in a more challenging direction.

Think about these possibilities:

- Freelance Makeup Artist for Print, TV, or Film
- Retail Specialist
- Distributor Representative
- Sales Consultant
- Student Instructor
- Professional Instructor
- School Administrator
- Retail Educator
- Retail Manager
- Industry Consultant
- Spa/Salon Manager
- Salon/Day Spa Owner
- Franchise Owner
- School/Academy Owner
- Events Coordinator
- Platform Artist
- Distributor/ Product Company
- Freelance Editorial / Professional Magazine

The list is endless! It is almost intimidating. But if you sit quietly with yourself and think about what you want to send out to the world, your answer will be crystal clear. Most of the time you already know when it is time to be moving on!

"And the day came when the risk to remain tight in a bud was more painful than the risk it took to blossom."
Anais Nin

Tips & Snips

Write, in order of preference, 3 career directions your desire:

Direction one:_____

Direction two:_____

Direction three:_____

CHANGE

Are you tired of doing the same old look on your client? Does he or she complain that they just can't do a thing with their hair? Then redesign your attitude this year for CHANGE! Starting with YOU!

It Starts With You

When was the last time you gave yourself a new look? Are you walking around with an old "do" expecting to change the look of a client's old "do"? Well, let's look in the mirror and understand that for us to convince our clients to change, we have to start with ourselves and BE the change. Take a few minutes to "be" a client and investigate your own options. Look at your best assets and try to bring forth a new you that exudes confidence. Step out of your box and try a fun crazy color placement that stimulates people to say, "WOW that looks great! Can we do something like that on me?"

Do this and you will instantly be doing some quick money making highlights.

Take Time for a LOOK BOOK Consultation

Pictures speak a thousand words. Grab your hairstyle books and begin showing your client looks that you feel will fit her bone structure, facial features, and lifestyle. Have her look with you and show you what she is comfortable with and what will not work. This is the one very overlooked skill that when professionals are too busy, seem to overlook. But the truth is, if you don't take the time to present new ideas, someone else will. Communication is the true key to a happy client. When you both visually agree on a look, your success is almost guaranteed.

Still Scared

Get with the program - this is 2007 and technology has never been better. There are many ways that you can get your client to see what they would look like in their new "do" by imaging. The fear of change can be reduced drastically with the power of the computer. Clients can now browse hairstyles and digitally see themselves in the latest looks, including color!

You can create a big event in your salon by hosting a party just by offering imaging! How fun is that? Do you know how many people want to change but just can't bear the thought of really making the change? A lot! People are uncomfortable with change. It is a human nature. So it is our professional duty to help them feel the fear and do it anyway.

You know they're going to love it. Client's are going to comment on it, and then guess what happens …yes, they bring you a friend!

Don't Forget to TEACH Them

Nothing is more frustrating to you as the designer of this great new look than to see your client out in public wearing your creation …backwards! We have seen it one too many times, the client leaves the salon looking and feeling marvelous only to see her hair out on the streets a complete mess, no shape, no style. Guess what? It is your disaster. Why? Because after all that work you put into it you didn't finish your job, and that was to TEACH your client HOW to work with the new "do". This is the single most important quality in a hairdresser that makes you stand out in front of all the rest. It is the time you give to your clients to ensure they know when they leave, how to style that masterpiece at home!

This is the opportunity that creates the bond between client and stylist. This is a time that you can capitalize on your retail sales. He or she simply must have those special products that you used on their head; otherwise it won't turn out the same at home.... Remember?

So help your clients make the change, you be the change!

To your success!

The Truth In The Mirror

WANT TO KEEP YOUR CLIENTS? TEACH THEM!

There is nothing worse than designing a hairstyle, which you know looks simply beautiful on your client, only to bump into that client out in public and see the hairstyle look embarrassingly awful. How many times have you heard your client say, "It looks great now, but when I do it, it doesn't look this way"? Or, "Could you come over to my house every morning to fix my hair?"

Many years ago, I learned the lesson of a lifetime that has become one of the biggest components to my growing business: give clients a great hairstyle and a shared experience, BUT ALSO TAKE THE TIME TO TEACH THEM HOW TO DO THEIR HAIR. I cannot begin to tell you how many referrals I have gotten from just that one very simple, often overlooked tactic.

I completely understand how busy we all get, but I highly encourage stylists to make it a priority to close the sale, and that means teaching the client how to care for their hair! How can you sell products without explaining and showing them how to use them effectively? Clients need to watch and listen as you demonstrate the purpose and function of the styling products as well as the use of the brush and dryer. Don't assume that everyone knows how to blow-dry his or her own hair. Clients are usually all thumbs when it comes to using our tools. If you don't believe me, just give your client the brush and dryer and tell them you want to make sure they know what to do, then watch what happens. You will see why, when you see them out in public, their hair doesn't resemble your original design!

A long time ago, I was sitting at a school function with four women, none who knew I was a hairdresser. The women were criticizing one of the board members. I overheard them say, "Look at her hair, she looks like Bozo the clown." This woman just happened to be one of my clients, and although she didn't look like Bozo when she left the salon, she did that day. I had failed as a stylist to teach her how to style her hair properly after I had given her a permanent wave. Had I taken the time to teach her what to do with her new perm, there would have been no rude comments. This is just one example of why we should remember to teach our clients; the big picture is that it truly makes you look creditable.

The rewards are endless when your client leaves the salon with a confident feeling and their confidence continues when they can duplicate your style again on their own. That fantastic feeling stays long after the service is over, and you gain even more respect as his/her personal stylist. Teaching your clients promotes a long-lasting relationship because it shows your concern about their appearance. So, if it is true that "Selling is Telling", then it's also true that "Teaching is Keeping"!

"The wisest mind has something yet to learn."
George Santayana

Tips & Snips

Today, what will you show your clients?

One: Product/Demo
Two: Tool Technique
Three: Ways to Style

CHAIR SIDE MANNERS

With the back to school madness upon us, it only seems appropriate to get our own backpack together with some mental tools and goals for approaching the coming season.

Fall is a very busy time for salon professionals. The holidays are near and the back to school rush is just beginning. This is a time when we can find ourselves overworked, drained of energy, and carelessly blowing out heads instead of consciously servicing our valued clients. The temptation is to just go through the motions and pray for an end to the long days. The reality is that we should be primed for the blessed and most profitable season we have all year.

One way to stay on track of your chair-side manners is to go back to the basics and consider the importance of a "client consultation." Remember when you first started out as a hairdresser? How much time did you spend on that new client? You asked her questions, listened attentively, perhaps you suggested a few new ideas of your own. Clients love that! It gives them a sense of clarity about what exactly they want. It also gives you a chance to get to know them and learn about their personality a little before you start to work with their hair. By opening yourself up and consulting with a client, you personalize the client experience and build a lasting connection.

Everyone could use a friendly reminder on the importance of a proper consultation, so let's remember the basics. Your main goal is to make the client relax, and help them find trust in you.

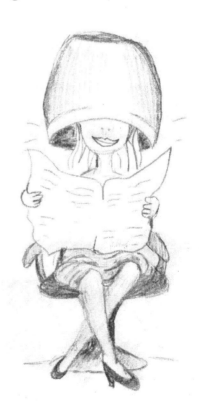

Here are 5 easy keys to remember:

1. Listen

Listen to what it is they are saying. Look in their eyes. Begin to ask questions about what they like and don't like about their hair, the type of life style they have, and how much time they plan to spend styling their hair.

2. Clarify

Clarify what it is they are saying. Repeat the statements they make, so they know you heard them and that you understand what they mean.

3. Suggest

Suggest a few ideas of your own. Even if they are not going to try something new today, you still planted the idea for them to think about in the future.

4. Get Permission

Get permission to do the idea. After you have both settled on what will be done, you still need their permission to do the service. Simply say again what you both agreed on.

5. *Act*

Begin the service with a smile! The best way to keep a client returning in your chair is to continually treat them to your best "chair side manners."

"Tell me and I forget; show me and I remember; involve me and I understand."

Unknown

Tips & Snips

Review:

One: LISTEN
Two: CLARIFY
Three: SUGGEST
Four: GET PERMISSION
Five: ACT

TIP, TIPPING, TIPPED...

"To give gratitude to; to give secrete information to; a hint; a warning; a tip of advice"

Let's Talk About Tips

As a hairdresser, we rely on tips. Our income levels vary for a stylist employed by a salon as well as a booth renter or independent contractor. A tip to us usually is the biggest form of a thank you when a good service is performed and the client is pleased with our work. But what about all the other tips we get as a bonus or benefit to our profession? How many times have you had clients in your chair give you a tip on a investment, a lead on a job for a friend, a piece of information on taxes, an insight to travel, a suggestion to help your business? We are surrounded by tips. Tips help us to grow and become fully human. Our profession has so many prosperous tips that we need to recognize and understand that we are being tipped all day long. Think about it, just say that you were struggling with needing a financial adviser for yourself, all you really have to do is mention a few times during the course of your day that you are in the market for some information, and before you know it, you have people recommend their uncle, their husband, neighbor etc. People love to help other people. For each client with which you build a rapport, after you talk about their hair needs, the conversation is usually about what's happening in each other's life. Our profession gives us access to EVERYTHING we need in life. We are so filled with tips, that we don't ever need to open up the yellow pages, hire a physiologist, find a date, or buy a how-to book. Whatever you're in the market for is right there in your chair.

Best Tip

One of the many best tips I have ever received was when a long time client of mine was starting up a hospital employee benefit program, and she was in the process of developing a newsletter for her clients. She new that at that time I was in the start-up process of my salon and she suggested that it might be a nice idea for my clients to receive a personal newsletter from me, about the salon happenings, tips, information, up-coming specials etc Although I never thought I could write, I threw it out there and it has since opened up a whole new world for me. The newsletter was an impressive way of communicating with my clients and they were excited to hear and experience all the new happenings of their "little but mighty" salon. . It also became a blueprint for my business for the year ahead. This ONE tip was the beginning of my new found love of writing. Since then, I went back to school to take journalism courses, and have written articles that have been published in many of our professional magazines and online. How could I have anticipated that my client's tip would inspire me to pursue this new direction?

Simple Steps To A Newsletter

1. Choose a format that you will keep consistent.

2. Use your salon logo, and incorporate fun graphics.

3. Use the 5 W"'s: "Who, What, Where, When, Why" when planning and writing about events.

4. Personalize your newsletter by featuring articles, quotes, recommendations about/from clients (and include their names).

5. Include a savings coupon for product or services (with a published expiration date).

6. Send it out with a regular frequency that you are comfortable with (monthly, quarterly, annually).

SELLING IS TELLING

Why is it that stylists don't like to recommend retail products? Is it that you fear rejection? Do you think the client won't be willing to pay a particular price for a certain shampoo or styling product? Well, think again! Selling retail is a big part of your service. It's your responsibility as a professional to recommend the proper products and tools to help your client duplicate the look they leave the salon with.

Show & Tell Technique

It is so simple to sell retail. You are merely telling them with a quick demonstration of how it is properly used. Think of it like when you were a child and had "Show and Tell" at school. As a stylist, you know what products work best on which hair types, so when you are in the process of styling the client's hair, just explain everything you are doing. Tell them what products you are using and why they need to continue using them.

Less Than A Minute

Taking the time to show your client a few techniques to make their styling at home easier will give your professionalism a high credibility. There is nothing a client wants more than to know how to keep his/her hairstyle looking as fabulous as when they left your chair. It only takes minutes out of your time to get your client to touch, smell, and experience the benefits of your retail products.

Let's Play

Prompting your client to handle the product is a great selling strategy. While he/she is in your chair, your products are always facing them and as you use each product you hand them the bottle, open it, take some out and put it in their hand. This way, they can listen to you talk and demonstrate, while they experience the touch and smell. It is incredible how the whole selling process comes to life. They learn about the product and feel more confident in its performance, therefore wanting to purchase it.

Make All Products Your Favorite

When you think about your favorite product, don't you just want everyone to know about it? When you're telling someone about a product, you get excited because you like what it does and how it makes your hair look, feel, and behave. Why not show that level of excitement with ALL of your products? Make them come alive with your personal testimony. Clients respect your opinion and expertise more than anyone, so next time you're trying to sell retail…just "show and tell".

"Gratitude unlocks the fullness of life."
Melody Beattie

Tips & Snips

What products will you tell your clients about?

Product one:_____

Product two:_____

Product three:_____

CONSTRUCTIVE CONVERSATION

Beware of who is in your chair! Day in and day out you carry on conversations with your clients and coworkers. Can you remember who or what you even talked about? Was it professional? Or was it gossip? Did you speak of beauty, or did you fall off track? Were you focused, or did you get caught in a mousetrap? Did you ever wonder at the end of the day *who* really was sitting in your chair? Think about how many people you come in contact with. You know most of them well - or at least you think you do.

Awkward Situations

But have you ever had a client catch you off guard? You know, that client who comes in every five weeks like clockwork, year after year. The one you have developed a nice friendly rapport with and then BAM! He throws you for a loop. He starts chasing you around your chair for "just one little kiss," knowing full well that you're married and he is too.

Or the client who has always been kind hearted, very calm, and sweet, and then one day comes in and is agitated, has got a new look in his eye, speaks in a whole different tone, and tells you that he doesn't know why, but lately he feels like killing someone - and it is just you and him in the salon!

You may not be able to circumvent those situations, but there are plenty of others that you can - if you stay focused on the professional aspects of the business and exercise tact and diplomacy when the conversation crosses the line.

Spies Among Us

I once had a new client call on the phone to set up an appointment, but when I asked who referred her, she said a name I didn't recognize. The woman showed up and seemed anxious, but I deal with many different personalities and I pride myself on being able to get along with all of them. Nonetheless, throughout the consultation she seemed familiar but I didn't know why. When we started the service I started with small talk to break the ice.

She began to ask lots of questions that weren't related to hair but were personal questions about me and my life. I was reluctant to answer her increasingly personal questions, yet I tried to remain warm and open in order to develop a new client relationship.

When the woman asked me if I had a boyfriend, I told her I was happily, recently taken. She told me she had a son, my age; I hinted that I knew a lot of single friends that might be interested, yet she continued to try to fix me up with her son. As the conversation became more uncomfortable, a weekly client came in and I introduced 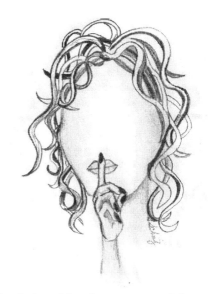 her to my new client. She joined in the conversation about my new boyfriend and commented that she wanted to meet him to see if he was good enough for me (you know your weekly ladies are always looking out for you). No sooner did she say that, when my boyfriend came in and just as I was about to introduce him to the ladies, he went right up to my new client and gave her a kiss and said "Hi Mom!"

These are just a few situations you may come across and I'm sure you have a few tales yourself. The point is that our career is colorful and part of our job is conversation and dealing with people from all walks of life. We need to pay attention to our clients' needs as well as maintain our own boundaries. It is important to have a firm grip on the relationships you build with clients. It's also good to trust your instincts but have good boundaries so that you can handle the awkward situations that are sure to arise.

Client challenges will forever be mysterious, just be on guard and on your best behavior. You may not really know who is sitting in your chair.

"One of the greatest pleasures of life is conversation."
Sydney Smith

Tips & Snips

Remember:

Always be Professional

Keep Conversation Simple

Listen More than Talk

Shaping And Draping

SUCCESSFULLY BRANDING YOUR SALON'S PERSONA

The salon industry is a people business full of all types of personalities, but what about your salon's personality? Are you clear about the image you are presenting to the public? In other words, how do you market your salon's style? Branding your salon gives your business an identity and helps build your reputation. It's a way for clients to quickly understand what your salon is all about.

Creating A Motto

Coming up with a motto is an excellent way to identify your salon and its focus. Start with an affirmation about the type of salon you are. Affirmations clarify your image and make a connection between your mindset and what you deliver on a day-to-day basis. It is the same as having a daily goal that you strive for that sets the foundation for your business.

At my salon, my motto is "Enhancing Your Total Self-Image is Our Business." Although I operate the salon alone with a part time assistant, I stay focused by keeping my energy high and referencing my motto in my day-to-day experiences. My motto sharpens my goal: to satisfy the client's individual taste with a made-to-order experience.

What's Your Niche?

There are all types of salons out there, from bargain basements to prestigious day spas. Each one has its own style of doing business. I'm convinced that clients come to us for the whole package.

- ✂ They come for the service.
- ✂ They admire the ambiance.
- ✂ They want convenience.
- ✂ They want variety and quality in the services they choose.
- ✂ They want to relax.

Although these qualities are important, the most important reason a client returns to us is for the FEELING OF COMFORT. Clients want to go to a salon that gives them a positive self-image but also makes it easy for them to express themselves. In order for a client to feel comfortable, they need to know what your salon is all about. Are you a place where everyone knows your name, or are you a quiet salon that reflects a formal setting? Quick-cut salons appeal to some and the royalty of day-spas appeal to others. It is all about the personality of the client and what they need. Your salon style validates who you are to the public.

Do An Inventory

Take a few minutes to think about how you present your salon. Do you have a motto? Do you carry a theme throughout your marketing? Would you visit your salon? Why? Why not? The style in which you present yourself is in direct proportion with how you conduct and maintain your business. The bonds between client and salon are built on trust, loyalty and shared life experiences that continue to grow after each visit.

The bottom line is that we are in a people business, and people respond to atmospheres that reflect their personalities. Our job is to create an environment that attracts the type of personality that will encourage our business to grow. A great gauge for your salon's success is when a client leaves with a smile and returns with a friend!

Branding My Salon

With my motto focused and a clear understanding of my clientele, I created a space reminiscent of an Italian Bistro. I adore cafés and wanted to create that feeling of relaxation and comfort you get when you are sitting in a café. My little-but-mighty salon has rich, energetic, yet soothing colors, wicker and iron chairs, cascading grapevines, and recessed display shelves with functional track lighting that enhances the sales of product. The salon gives a lighthearted feeling and a sense of unity and comfort with oneself. Clients enjoy being connected to a place where they can express themselves and I encourage that feeling by adapting to each client's personality. This has been the tapestry and the nature of the success in my business.

Using the "bistro theme," virtually all my marketing materials carry a restaurant "flavor". From the bunch of grapes incorporated into the salon name to the menu of services with offerings listed by course, the

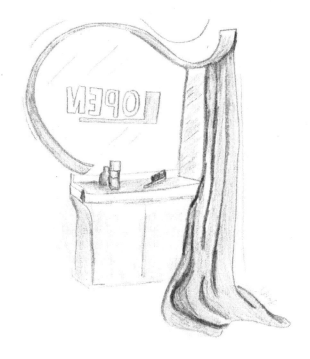

theme is carried throughout the salon. This marketing objective delivers a comfortable yet creative message, and leaves unlimited possibilities for new materials.

No matter what your salon's "persona" is, if it is clearly connected to the essence of your spirit, your clients will be eager to return again and again.

Imagine!

Tips & Snips

Write your personal mission statement:

_____

_____

_____

_____

_____

IT PAYS TO BE ORGANIZED

There are only three types of people in this world: people who plan to fail, people who fail to plan, and people who plan and succeed. Which one will *you* be this year?

How many times have you told yourself on December 31st that your New Year's resolution this year would be to stay focused on your business and be organized? That this will be the year you clean out your file cabinet and start fresh? Well, that is exactly what you must do if you want a successful business and reduce stress.

It all starts with a plan. You need to begin your New Year with a focus - a blueprint of your year ahead for all the things you want to accomplish. You must put it in writing either in calendar form or in a structured sequence; some way that allows you to view it often, so that you can stay on track of your goals.

Your plan should be extremely detailed to make it crystal clear to everyone the plan for the salon's success. Planning is vital for the success of your year, because it is a constant reminder that you always have something to be working on. The "what next" attitude becomes exciting, not only for you and your staff but for clients as well. Take it a step further and create a calendar of events for clients, too!

Knowing what to do takes the guesswork out of your day. Having a blueprint of your year ahead also is an excellent way to review your past year in order to see what worked and what didn't. All you need is a piece of paper, a pen, and your imagination. Incorporating a well-organized plan for your year ahead opens up a world of opportunity for your future.

"For the happiest life, days should be rigorously planned,
nights left open to chance."

Mignon Mclaughlin

Tips & Snips

Write three ways to organize your year ahead:

1st way:_____

2nd way:_____

3rd way:_____

HELPING HANDS

They say that we, as salon professionals, have the power to touch people and transform lives. That statement alone is the most honorable achievement any career could offer. Our profession is about truly enhancing the morale of other people. The day-to-day work of beauty professionals develops into heartfelt relationships where we feel connected and are committed to helping others face some of the misfortunate challenges that may arise in their personal lives. This industry is about the people, making them look and feel magnificent no matter what is going on in their life.

A Call To Duty

There comes a time when people need big help. Who better to rise to the occasion than you, your salon or your peers? Putting your efforts in supporting programs such as Brest Cancer Awareness, Cut it Out programs, helping the homeless, donating to Katrina or just your support to a heartfelt cause will pay off to you more than any amount of money you could ever make. Coming together as a team of supporters allows you to become involved in a spiritual community of blessing those less fortune than yourself.

You learn to place enormous value on your own personal health and lifestyle and create a positive force into the lives of others. Your support goes far beyond a monetary donation. What you receive emotionally will well exceed what you gave out of your pocket or of your time. Knowing that you personally helped enhance the quality of someone else's existence is the true meaning of support.

The Good News

How do you feel when you pick up a magazine or the paper and you read an article about an organization or company that has just raised $1 Million dollars by offering their personal services to help out some little child whom was very ill, or a family who was destitute and your salon pulled together and raised enough money to get some of their needs met? Maybe your stylist committed herself to the Avon Brest Cancer 3 day walk and you had a supporting donation box to remind all the clients of her challenge and help with encouragement. These are the stories that need to be told. This is the good news that people of all ages like to read and hear about. It is uncanny the publicity that you will receive from being a part of positive programs that help to celebrate the lives and well being of others.

Let's Make Some Noise

Besides the power to affect people with the united force of dedication, you also receive the big benefit of impact marketing. People like it when they hear or see what you are made of. If your salon gets involved and your community, or the newspaper even industry related publications find out… they all want to capture your story and share what Good you're doing and how it is affecting others.

COSMETOLOGY IS BOOMING!

Our industry is booming with opportunities that are filled with options, flexibility, and a grand potential to make an impressive living.

According to occupational handbooks, cosmetology is expected to grow faster than average, offering work in all capacities from extreme to in-between success. Overall employment for personal appearance workers is projected to grow through 2012, because of increasing population, incomes, and demand for personal appearance services.

Trained Professionals Facts

According to the U.S. Department of Labor, barbers, cosmetologists, and other personal appearance workers held about 754,000 jobs in 2002. Of these, barbers, hairdressers, hairstylists, and cosmetologists held 651,000 jobs; manicurists and pedicurists, 51,000; skin care specialists, 25,000; and shampoo staff, 25,000.

Almost half of all barbers, cosmetologists, and other beauty professionals are self-employed. Many own their own salon, but a growing number lease booth space or a chair from the salon's owner.

According to a 2000 National Accrediting Commission of Cosmetology Arts and Science (NACCAS) report, in 1999 there were 297,000 salons in the U.S. and 1,286,00 licensed cosmetologists. More than either the number of elementary school teachers or lawyers. This figure includes people who are licensed but not currently practicing.

The typical salon is a small, full-service salon with five stations, two or three full-time professionals, and one part-time professional. Salon owners report an average of 174 clients per week.

- ✂ 70% of salon owners classified their salon as a full-service salon, 13% as a hair cutting salons, 4% as a nail salon, and 9% as a barbershop.

- ✂ 60% of salon employees work full time, 29% are part time (20-35 hours), and 11% are low time (less than 20 hours).

- ✂ The average salon income, including tips,

appears to be at about $18.50/hour.

✂   While manicurists are currently only 20% of
the current industry employee base, some
21% of anticipated vacancies are for
professionals with those skills.

(Source: National Accrediting Commissions of Cosmetology
Arts and Sciences (NACCAS)-"Job Demand in the
Cosmetology Industry, 2003")

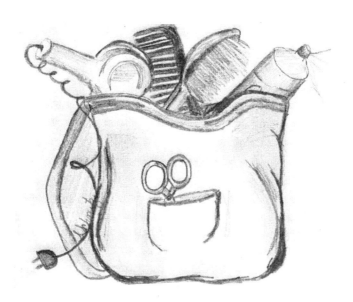

Earnings Potential

The U.S. Bureau of Labor statistics has projected that the number of jobs in cosmetology will increase by 100% by 2008.

Job openings will arise from the need to replace workers who transfer to other occupations or retire, or leave the labor force for other reasons. The competition in this industry is expected to be intense, as applicants compete with a large pool of licensed and experienced cosmetologists who are highly educated from the advanced training received at beauty schools today.

The 1999 Occupational Handbook from the U.S. Department of Labor estimated the average entry-level salary for cosmetologists to be $15, 150.

According to the U.S. Department of Labor "Median annual earnings in 2000 for salaried hairdressers, hairstylists, and cosmetologists, including tips and commission, were $17,660. The middle 50 percent earned between $14,000 and $23,910. The lowest 10 percent earned less than $12,280 and the highest 10 percent earned more than $33,220. Median annual earnings were $17,620 in beauty shops and $17,570 in department stores."

Other Factors

There are a number of factors that determine the total income for cosmetologists, barbers, and other beauty professionals. Depending on your personal success and desire, your income is determined by your career decisions. There are many cosmetologist who make over $100,000 annually. They simply apply themselves and have found the correct 'establishment' in which to perform their trade. Factors may include the location of a salon, the number of hours worked, the clients' tipping habits, and the method by which they are paid (i.e., salary, commission, compensation for retail products sold, client retention, potential growth scale, etc.) There are many opportunities in the beauty industry to advance your career and further your income options. This career is mobile.

Some salons offer paid vacations and medical benefits, but many self-employed and part-time workers in this occupation do not enjoy these benefits. These are things to consider when selecting your chosen direction.

(Source: U.S. Department of Labor-Bureau of Labor Statistics-Occupational Outlook Handbook-Barbers, Cosmetologists, and other Personal Appearance Workers-Earnings http: //ststs.bls.gov/oco/ocos/169.htm)

The best objective for a cosmetologist is to strive to become a well -rounded professional, providing a broad range of services.

Pump It Up!

CLIENT APPRECIATION: SAY IT OUT LOUD!

As I approach the madness of the holidays, I feel it's important to take a few minutes to sit and think about the many blessings of our industry.

Thanksgiving is a time of year to remind us of the wonderful people in our lives, both professionally and personally. It is also a time to reflect on the everyday treasures that we don't even realize are truly gifts. One very overlooked blessing is the nature of our profession. We are in an industry that is all about being positive. Our main mission is to make people look and feel magnificent. Think about that for a moment. We help our clients see their own personal beauty. Through our artistry, we visualize, we create, and we let our inspiration flow. We get to talk about life issues, help clients solve their problems, and sometimes we even get to solve our own. There is no need to have to pick up the paper; we get the entire outside world news right in our chair. Being in the beauty industry allows us to dress fashionably, listen to upbeat music, and have the freedom to express ourselves. All this, and we get PAID highly for doing it. Have you yet to find another career that is so fulfilling personally and professionally? So my fellow stylist, it is time to give THANKS this season to the people who make this industry survive…our clients.

Create A Client-Appreciation Event

How can you say thank you? There are many ways to show your appreciation to your clients. One exciting idea is to host a client-appreciation bash! Holding an event like this once year lets clients get together in a fun atmosphere and makes them feel special! Yes, it can be a little costly, but the rewards far outweigh the expense. Begin your client appreciation party planning with a few basics:

Create A Theme

Use your theme throughout your decorating and promotional materials.

Example: Groovy 60's & 70's: use peace signs, flower power, and smiley faces throughout the salon. Have dripping candles on all the tables with incense burning. Make tablecloths out of old bandannas, and centerpieces with tissue paper flowers.

Plan A Menu

Plan your menu around the theme and serve foods that will complement your theme. You can also ask your clients to bring a community dish so they can feel part of the event and can use their own creativity. This will also help to keep costs down and add to the fun.

Example: fondue, wild mushrooms, brownies, Boone's Farm Wine, keg beer, etc.

Entertainment

You cannot have a party without music. Everybody has a client in his or her list that knows someone in a band or plays the guitar or may even be a DJ. Start asking around. You will be surprised at how many talented people you have right in your chair. You can work out the payment in trade or simply take on the cost yourself.

Play Games

Parties are more memorable when you break up the evening with games.

Example: Sticking with the theme of the party, "name the pet rock" contest; give it away as a prize. TV and music trivia of that era is fun. And you can network with all of your clients who own businesses and get promotional (stuff) donated for prizes. That way you are including more people in on the event and promoting them as well.

Thank Everyone

Let's face it; you wouldn't have a business without your faithful clients. Some will always drive you crazy; some will always touch your heart. But the one thing that keeps our industry going is the client. Take a moment in the evening to thank everyone for his or her continual patronage – this shows that you appreciate their friendship as well as their business.

Have Fun!

"Life should be lived as play!"

Plato

Tips & Snips

Plan your event:

Where:_____

When:_____

What:_____

WHAT IS TREND?

What is your answer when a client asks you..."What's the latest trend?" Do you scramble to identify the latest styles? Think of the last magazine you thumbed through for a quick tip you can give to your client? Or do you keep up with the current direction of the hair and fashion world so that you can help your client express himself or herself more abundantly?

Every decade brings with it a new flair for trends. If you can recall back, you can see how trends set a tone for their era of time. Trends are simply a fresh and timely approach to any industry. In the hair industry we often refer to trends by certain celebrities that set the styles, or by magazines that help the public view fashion.

Think back to the '70s. It was a time of the famous Farrah Fawcett feathers that everyone desired. Then came the big teased out, wild perms, with the sky high mall bangs of the '80s (thank God that's over) and to really throw us off, the trends then changed to super sleek, poker-straight hair for the '90s. These are just a few examples of how we relate to trends. Fashion sets a tone and direction that everyone can follow.

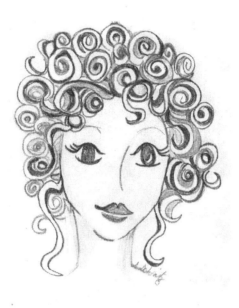

But do all trends really look good on everyone? No. A trend is the current look created for the season. It isn't meant for everyone to wear. It is the artist's vision for a fresh look. A new approach to an old technique perhaps, or a creation inspired by the artist's emotion.

Today, with the open palette of expression and freedom of style, the best advice you can give to your clients on trends is that a trend is what defines their image. It is what works for them, with their bone structure, their facial features, and their lifestyle. It is a hairstyle or fashion statement that makes them feel fabulous.

Trends come and go in the beauty industry. You just have to be open to trying out a few new techniques that help to enhance their own personal look.

Timeless "Trends"

✂ Bangs, yes, all different sexy lengths of soft bangs that frame the face, open the eyes, and give a fresh feeling to hair.

✂ Curls, lots of textures to be bouncing around, from tight corkscrew locks to carefree flowing waves.

✂ Color, no fear here, please. Open your mind to the wonderful world of individual expression of color. No rules.

✂ Makeup, don't forget to define your clients' self-image with the dramatic shades of color for that season.

"What we see depends mainly on what we look for."
John Lubbock

Tips & Snips

Get the News:

1. Industry Magazine:_____

2. Take a Class:_____

3. Go Online:_____

CREATIVE BUSINESS: BARTERING FOR SERVICES

We encounter people everyday with whom we can do business and there are ways to be creative and build great business relationships at the same time. One way to foster new relationships is by bartering for services. Ever imagine exchanging a haircut for a sump pump installation, or giving someone a perm in exchange for lawn services? Bartering allows your creative spirit and business sense to open up new avenues for you to build your trade.

No Money Involved

The biggest advantage of bartering is that there's no money required up front - and let's face it, we all like a good deal. Not having to go into your pocketbook once in awhile is kind of sweet. You just have to know how to keep the score even so no one feels slighted.

I remember one time, the carpenter husband of a very good client of mine had an idea for my salon (to make recessed shelving for my retail center), but at the time I wasn't in a financial situation to afford to pay for his work. My client told me not to worry. We would exchange my hair services for her husband's carpentry work. She kept a log of the monetary value of my services and the value of his work and we shook hands. It was a wonderful exchange that benefited both of us and another reason to count the blessings in life.

Keep It Simple

Most bartering exchanges in salons are informal. They range from simple, one-time agreements to more complicated, ongoing swaps. Unfortunately, there are occasions when one trader is looking for even more than you bartered for. That is when you run the risk of ending a relationship instead of building one. That's why you need to keep all swaps clear.

You can also expand the bartering field to include friends and members of your family, provided that they are willing to trade services as well. If a client is looking for home repairs, I let them know that my husband can fix anything, and then we work out a trade for 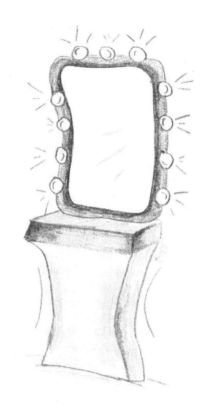 his services. If not, I recommend many of my other clients who do that type of work. That is the intertwined connection beauty professionals have with the world and it is a powerful business tool.

Just Ask

When it comes to bartering, I'm not shy. If a client has something I want, I do not hesitate to try and work out a deal. A client of mine just got her esthetician license and now does facials. Now I cut and color her hair in exchange for her wonderful facials. I feel good about that barter and so does she. We both have agreed that there will be no money exchanged, just services.

Keeping Track - Bartering Consultation

To determine a fair price, both parties need to determine what they would charge for the bartered service, whether it is a plumbing job or a new coat of paint or in my case, hair services. On my end, I give the person I'm bartering with a credit for the amount of my services. I keep a record of the amount in a book and each time they come in, I make a deduction until they've used up the total amount of the trade. Spending one-on-one time with the trader will help clarify the terms of the barter. I call this the consultation technique, which involves the following steps: Listen, Clarify, Suggest, Get Permission and Act.

- ✂ Listen to what you both need.
- ✂ Clarify what you both heard.
- ✂ Make suggestions on what you're not comfortable with.
- ✂ Get permission from the other bartering party to do the service and at what price.
- ✂ Then ACT on it!

Be Aware

Well-detailed records have another bonus: lowering the stress level that may arise during tax time. Not having to put money up front is definitely a bartering bonus, but do keep in mind that Uncle Sam will want to collect his share come April 15. Barter and cash transactions are the same in the eyes of the Internal Revenue Service. So just keep that in mind as you trade in your baloney sandwich at the lunch table for your friend's peanut butter and jelly.

Bartering is a great way to network your business, and it will foster good will in your community.

"Obstacles are those frightful things you see when you take your eyes off the goals."

Unknown

Tips & Snips

What services do you need?

_____

_____

_____

_____

_____

REAL BEAUTY

There was an age when a woman's physical beauty was considered her most prized possession. Today, however, women define beauty more in terms of how they feel and less in terms of how they look. It is great that women are getting more in touch with their authentic beauty.

Beauty is complex. Beauty is broad. Beauty is different in different times of our lives. It is self-realization, it is an internal light, a spiritual radiance that all women have, but many forget to embrace. Beauty comes from within. It comes from that sacred place in your soul that reminds you of your worthiness on this planet.

Beauty is simplicity. The simple things in life that change the way you view your world. Beauty is accepting yourself as you are today and embracing the mirror with pride. Beauty is in loving yourself for all that you are and all that you are going to be. It allows you to be kind to yourself, to honor your true feelings and your needs. Beauty is love - love of self, an ancient beauty secret available to all of us.

Let's face it. We can't all look like movie stars, but each of us can look like our BEST selves. The way to achieve the real essence of beauty is by beginning to realize that through personal transformations - whether in lifestyle or in appearance - our beauty will always come from the true work of spiritual growth.

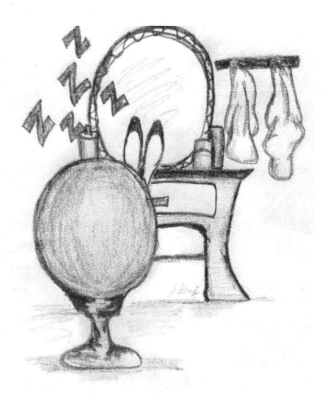

Beauty Treatments For Your Soul

Today offers a multitude of beauty treatments. The rising trends of spas that provide the consumer with any type of beauty enhancers and products are one way to jump-start your beauty regime. Or you can take an alternative approach and seek out what works for you. For some people this means joining a class, whether it is yoga, art, or an academic course at a local college. For others, it may be learning how to sit still, to be O.K. with silence so that you can hear your own inner voice.

Create Time For Yourself

To help develop your inner beauty, pencil yourself in your date book. Make a commitment to yourself every day to do the necessary things that make you feel energized or relaxed, even if it means you have to get up early or stay up late. Carve out that time to indulge in a great book or a good workout, or simply to sip your favorite beverage.

Love Yourself

Loving yourself unconditionally is the best beauty

treatment you ever will have. It is not conceited. People who love themselves take pride in their appearance and their health. They honor their spirits with loving gestures and celebrate how marvelous they can be. They live in gratitude and know the importance of balance. Because of their love for themselves, they treat everyone they meet with that same loving feeling. Loving yourself is the key to confidence. Self-confidence mixed with an optimistic attitude and a dash of enthusiasm will help you maintain healthy thoughts.

Passion

Having a passion for what you desire and a solid hope for your future is a loving and beautiful gesture. Passion is contagious. It's that driving force that keeps you alive. LOVE YOURSELF! BE PASSIONATE! MAKE TIME! These three ingredients create the perfect makeup for a beautiful face. Try it and you'll be certain to make the right connection to your mind, to your body, and to your soul.

"The door of the human heart can only be opened from the inside."

Unknown

Tips & Snips

Write three nice things you will do for yourself:

1. _____

2. _____

3. _____

NETWORKING! A POSITIVE PAYOFF

Network! Network! Network! That is what our business thrives on. Are you a small business with a big dream? Do you struggle to find new, innovative ways to keep your business personal, as well as profitable? Well, help is in your chair. That's right, in your chair. The clients that you see every day are your links to your future. It's called networking - networking with people - human contacts - the ones we have every single day. Our business is filled with opportunities to connect with people who can help us achieve our goals, and at the same time help them to reach theirs. Our industry sets the stage for personal one-on-one contact that allows all types of business transactions to occur.

It is all about the "web". The networking web that you already have started, sitting right in your chair. Think of your business behind the chair as if it were a gigantic spider web, with all of the people that you come in contact with being the intersecting threads of your web. Now, each one of these threads (clients) are the crossing lines to another thread, (i.e., friend, cousin, aunt, neighbor) creating yet another connection, and so on, and so on. The end result is that you, the spider, will continue to build your web by connecting people together and help them to build their own web, personal or professional.

You actually network all day long; you just haven't put it to use yet. Networking provides you with the personal touch you need to create relationships that are the fundamentals of being a smart business owner, no matter how big or small your establishment.

I'm an independent salon owner and networking is the way I do business. It has been an excellent way for me to promote and maintain a good rapport with my existing clients. I believe in connecting with people, so I find creative ways to network. One way that I found to network was through all my clients' businesses. Last fall I decided to join together with all my willing clients who owned small businesses and hold a Fall Festival. This was one of the most rewarding experiences I have ever had in all the years of doing business. It was a real win-win across the board for everyone who participated. There were ten to fifteen booths ranging from insurance agents to wine tasting, to crafts. Everyone was a client. We had a motivational speaker, a massage therapist, Mary Kay Cosmetics, even a songwriter/singer who entertained us all day long. The event was a smash hit. There was food prepared by a client who has a catering business, face painting networked through all of the clients' teenage children. We even played a version of the "Dating Game", with prizes and giveaways.

People were strolling the big yellow tent in amazement, realizing that there were so many people they knew just from patronizing the salon. The exchange of business cards and newfound friendships was a fantastic sight to behold, but the real highlight of that day was when I stepped back for a few moments and realized that those grounds were filled with tons of people, and those people were not strangers; they were all a part of the ever-reaching web of clients that I have serviced over the years. Networking is a positive payoff. It is made up of the tiny threads that weave into the fabric of our lives, both professionally and personally.

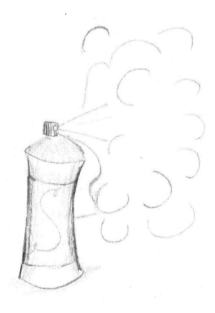

"Ideas are funny little things, they don't work unless you do."
Unknown

Tips & Snips

List three people or businesses you can network with:

1. _____

2. _____

3. _____

LET'S GO DO IT!

Fun, Fresh ways to Build your Empire!

- ✂ Create a Newsletter
- ✂ Design a big sign: "Want A Free Hair Cut? Ask Me How"... Mirror talkers
- ✂ Flyer with a special savings
- ✂ Get involved in church activities
- ✂ Ladies day out, Fashion shows
- ✂ Donations to charitable causes (i.e. a gift basket w/ service coupon and hair products)
- ✂ Go to schools and advertise Dance Up-do specials with unique package deal
- ✂ Teacher appreciation day
- ✂ Employee appreciation day @ local banks/ convenience stores
- ✂ Client appreciation day
- ✂ Capture business while sitting at your child's sporting events - ask if you can put out flyers
- ✂ Design a yearly calendar highlighting every month with an event or specials
- ✂ Create a punch card for haircuts (i.e. punch x # of cuts, get one half-off).

- ✂ Create a punch card for products – once all $$ on card for purchases are filled, get % discount or free product

- ✂ Publish in salon news magazine - inventive incentive program

- ✂ Host events, such as Open House, Cut-a-thons, Mothers Day In, Teen parties

- ✂ Host events with Guest Speakers on topics such as Health, Fashion, Makeup, Spirituality, Business/Marketing

- ✂ Network with your clients to host joint events

- ✂ Have a photo shoot

- ✂ Create a survey to find out what your clients want and need from you (and what they appreciate about your existing salon/services)

- ✂ Create a recipe book of your clients' favorite dishes, and then use it for a fund-raiser for a school or charity

- ✂ Host a million-dollar hair year. Give lottery tickets to the first 50 clients

- ✂ Host client contests, such as "Write an entry about why your mother should win a free day of beauty"

- ✂ Offer a free neck massage or eyebrow wax with any chemical service

- ✂ Host a client appreciation party – see "Big Bash", published in American Salon Magazine!

- ✂ Host a backyard "Festival". NETWORK with all your clients and create your own festival, including a "Dating game", face painting, music, guest speakers, vendors (team up with home party consultants), giveaways, wine tasting, raffles. Have plenty of prize opportunities

- ✂ Invent themes for Festivals: Bonfire in the Fall, Groovy Night (60's & 70's), Mad Hatter's Tea Party!

- ✂ Send cards to your clients: Thank you, birthday, sympathy, get-well, just thinking of you, encouragement, congratulations – include a personal note.

- ✂ Donate or participate in a raffle for anything!

- ✂ Are you my client of the month? Reward a special client with a gift certificate to the movies or a free service for being supportive

- ✂ READ industry related magazines, online articles, talk to your peers, but most of all…

Refer to your personal pocket coach *"As The Chair Turns… Tips and Snips of Advice for Your Journey Behind the Chair."*

HOLIDAY MADNESS

It's that time of year again! The pressure is on the way! Clients are talking about it. Kids are giving you their wish lists. The stores are decorated, the music is playing, and the stress of the wonderful time of year begins. The Holidays!

Although this is supposed to be a joyous time of year, for some reason the spirit often gets robbed - stolen by all the duties that you have to do in order to get through it all. You're booked solid for weeks, clients from the past suddenly call you for a "do", existing clients forgot to pre-book for the holidays, and you feel compelled to get them in, so, what do you do? You work longer hours, come in early, stay late, shop at midnight, eat on the run, fill yourself up with unhealthy foods, drink lots of fattening coffee drinks, and play super hairdresser, super mom, and super mate to your partner. It's crazy!

But if you want to grab hold of this season, and truly ENJOY what it is supposed to be all about, then do yourself a favor and try to change your old habits with a fresh approach so that you can sit calmly with your family and friends and embrace the season with love instead of frustration.

Breathe Deeply

First and foremost, take a deep breath, now exhale, another, now exhale even bigger, now exhale. Start each and every day by detoxifying your mind. With all that we hear each day, we need to detoxify yesterday's events. Try to not bring what happened yesterday into today. It's gone, and today is a brand new day to enjoy.

Get Up Early

Yes, that's right, set your alarm 45 minutes early so that you can *take time out* just for you - to get your mind, body, and spirit all on the same page of life. This is one of the healthiest things you can do for yourself in order to keep your sanity and to get in touch with your inner self (which is constantly lost by giving it all away every day to your clients and to your family). So give yourself a big gift this year, the gift of taking care of *you*.

Sit Still

You can! Just sit there quietly and be there. No TV, no radio, no one talking, just you and your world. Peace is worth millions. To just sit with yourself gives you the opportunity to think, and with all that you have to listen to, it allows you to listen only to your inner self for a few minutes.

Stretch

Move around for a few minutes. This doesn't mean you have to do an hour-long workout, but get your body moving by taking a moment to untangle. Think about how you stand all day and the small radius of movements that you have. We need to unlock ourselves so that we're not so stiff. So STRETCH! Try a 15-minute yoga tape in the morning - it will start your day with the vital positive energy you require in order to get through all those clients.

Eat Breakfast

Try it! Eating a healthy breakfast is a powerful way to start your day off in the right direction. No time? Try incorporating a high protein drink instead of a latte. You will save time, lots of money and create more healthy energy for yourself.

Take Vitamins

Because of the fast pace we live, and the toxic environment in which we work, we need to replenish all the nutrition we are losing daily. Start by taking a multi-vitamin and then after the holidays, give yourself the gift of health and go to a nutritionist and have an assessment. It is worth the effort to find out your health needs.

Pencil Yourself In

That's right! Pencil yourself in the books. Make sure you allow yourself time for your haircut and color, for your nail appointment or facial, and for your lunch date with old friends. It all sounds too good to be true, but if you just try to take 45 minutes each day to do these little things for yourself as well as pencil yourself into your schedule, you will feel so much better about the stress of the holidays because you allowed yourself the *personal time* that you desperately need in order to be productive during this wonderful time of the year! May this season bring to all of you blessed health and peace in you hearts.

"If you want to put the world right, start with yourself."
Unknown

Tips & Snips

Write three ways to prepare for the busy season:

1. _____

2. _____

3. _____

"SANTA CLAUSE IS COMING TO TOWN"

Are You Ready?

The Holidays are near. The department stores are prepared by loading up on gift-buying ideas for the happy shopper. They know how and when to capitalize on one of the biggest money making times of the year. Are YOU ready?

Salons across the country can enjoy more profitability at this time of year than any other by simply positioning themselves and their staff to "SELL MORE RETAIL". There is a 40% to 50% profit margin to be gained by selling retail products. It is one of the easiest times of the year because everyone is in the mood to spend money and shop till they drop. You can recoup a lot of your loss income by preparing your salon for the most wonderful time of the year.

Silver Bells

Create the spirit of holiday shopping and the gift-buying adventure by providing a festive shopping atmosphere. Decorate tastefully, choose a variety of Christmas music, and place signs to direct your clients to your products. Customers want that warm, inviting feeling to alter their buying experience. Everyone is forever walking around aimlessly or on a mission when the holidays are near, and setting the tone helps to entice the customer to relax and enjoy their shopping in your salon. When you have the proper environment, people will want to stay awhile and spend money. Offer ways to invite them to shop, by having a welcome table with refreshments and perhaps a flyer with all your gift packages listed so they can tour your retail area and go through each display. The idea is to give them a reason to hang out.

Selling Success

It is a proven fact that you will retain over 90% of your clients when they purchase professional products from you. Your clients want you to recommend your product choices to them. They need to understand the value of what the products can do for them at home as well as when they leave the salon. This builds credibility as a professional.

If you're not selling professional products to them, they will purchase elsewhere. Why let that happen? This is a profitable time; all you need is the energy to prepare your salon with great promotions and holiday ideas that create sales.

12 Days of Christmas "IDEAS"

- Capture your clients' attention with offers that they cannot resist
- Create signs that have a solid offer
- Prepare pre-packaged gift baskets
- Hold a VIP day
- Have an "Open House" every week
- Advertise a "Private Holiday Sale"
- Highlight a featured item
- Send postcards that offer Holiday product gifts at 20% off
- Offer a product coupon with next visit

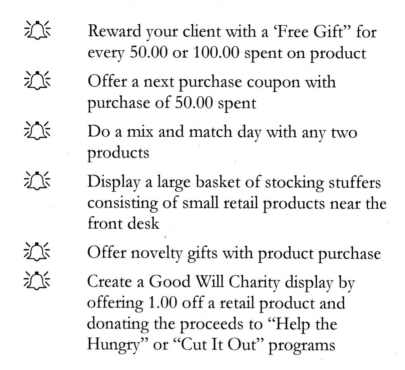

- Reward your client with a 'Free Gift" for every 50.00 or 100.00 spent on product

- Offer a next purchase coupon with purchase of 50.00 spent

- Do a mix and match day with any two products

- Display a large basket of stocking stuffers consisting of small retail products near the front desk

- Offer novelty gifts with product purchase

- Create a Good Will Charity display by offering 1.00 off a retail product and donating the proceeds to "Help the Hungry" or "Cut It Out" programs

One of the most winning selling techniques used in the sale of any product is the proper use of language. If you position your marketing to be eye catching as well as emotionally driven you are almost guaranteed to have a jolly Christmas season. Using enticing words on signs or displays lures your customer to want to experience the feeling implied by the description of the product. Examples: "Treat Yourself Right", "Fantasy Hair", "Sexy Lips", Age Defying" "Timeless Beauty".

Words play an important role in creating a mood for the client to purchase. When trying to up-sell a product, incorporate verbiage that will inspire an emotion. Customers want to feel what the product can do for them as well as the performance aspect that the product offers.

Santa's Little Helpers

REMEMBER THESE WORDS… Touch it, Smell It, Feel it, Buy it!

- ✂ Products need to be touchable
- ✂ Use effective language on signs or displays
- ✂ Keep well-stocked shelves
- ✂ Have a featured item of the week
- ✂ HELP them purchase

Wishing you A Merry Christmas, and a profitable and healthy New Year!

Tease It To New Heights

SOLO VERSES SALON: WEIGHING OUT THE DIFFERENCE

Are you ready to take the big leap and open the doors of freedom and independence? Or do you like the comfort of knowing you can depend on co- workers and salon management to keep you going? What's right for you?

Both journeys allow for different experiences that provide necessary knowledge that supports the passion for your career. In your first few years you need certain aspects of salon life to fully understand the way the business is run. The people that you work with are also your mentors, and educators that help shape and polish your skills that you will always take with you in your quest to discover your own style of being a beauty professional. Without salon experience, you would truly be missing out on an abundance of wisdom and day-to-day involvement that is crucial to the growth of a newborn professional. Those first few years can give you insight to new horizons, career choices, and networking opportunities that lead you to the next level and give you a foundation upon which to grow.

Structure

Everyone works more proficiently with a little structure. It sets the tone with a system in place that everyone is expected to follow. Structure works well to get a team to work together as well as providing rules and guidelines. Without it, everyone creates his or her own set of rules, the salon atmosphere is unmanageable, and the salon becomes permeated with confusion and negativity. So if you understand the value of structure, your salon life can be a great experience for you. One you can use as a blueprint for the future. Or, if you are a very disciplined and organized person, this may not be an issue for you.

Communication Skills

For those of you who are still in the developmental phase of your career, working in a salon is an excellent way to watch, listen and learn creative ways to handle all the different personalities you will encounter. It is also a great way for you to view how to approach people with confidence, and how to develop your retail sales offering to your clients. Communication is the biggest tool you use everyday, and without developing this skill you will have a very hard time in this business. Learning how to talk with your clients and peers takes constant and consistent effort in order to feel confident when handling personality differences. Remember, our business is a people business first, so you have to become comfortable with all age groups. The success of your business relies not only in your craft, but also in your personal style with people.

Paperwork/Bookkeeping

Having someone do all the behind the scenes work is a gift to hairdressers. By nature we are artists, and paperwork really doesn't interest us. If you are a "let me create and go" kind of person, then working in the salon is great for you. Your only paper responsibility is to yourself to know what you made for the day. On the other hand, if that is not an issue for you and you feel confident handling all the paperwork that goes with running a salon, you enjoy the numbers and figures of the business, are proficient in keeping good records, and set consistent strategies for growth, then being independent can work out well for you.

Progressive Growth

The beauty industry is extremely progressive, and if you plan on creating a life for yourself out of your investment, then prepare yourself for lifelong learning.

Change is the word that comes to mind when you are in this business, and you need to be able to move forward in order to stay with the times.

Working in a salon environment opens the doors to keeping up with the latest trends and techniques because you are around a variety of co-workers who share with you their personal styles and techniques. Working with a combination of people with different styles offers inspiration and influences you to become more creative with your own work…not to mention the fact that a little competition never hurt anyone. It keeps you on your path and helps you to discover your own uniqueness.

Being independent, you must be your own motivator and be able to know how to get inspiration. Your intuition is developed over time, but in the meantime, you still require stimulation to keep your energy high, especially when you are working alone. Maintaining a level of professional skills demands continual education, and your success is determined by how well you keep your mental, spiritual and professional image alive.

Challenge/Freedom

It is only natural for people to want to grow and feel in control of their lives. Isn't that the goal? To be able to learn as you go and move on to the next challenge. We all desire the freedom to express ourselves in our own way, which is one reason we want to go solo. But like everything else in life, we need certain aspects of experiences that give to us the necessary tools to withstand all of the challenges that arise when we are on our own. Time, people, environment, and shared common interest all play a key role in the confidence you need to become an independent.

No matter what path you choose, your success is what you believe in.

WHERE ARE MY CLIENTS?

Did you ever wonder why you haven't seen Mr. Jones in awhile? You gave him a great haircut, you provided him with superior service, your salon was neat and tidy, your conversation was flowing, and he looked like he left your chair very happy. But after a few months you noticed he hasn't returned. "What happened?" you ask yourself. I performed every aspect of my professional knowledge on Mr. Jones. Why did he choose not to return to me? These questions will come up and you may never learn the answers.

Never Stop Building Your Business

If there is one certain thing in this business, it's that clients come and go. You must always be building your business. It is a daily thought process to continue to replenish and rebuild your clientele. There is an old saying that you can take with you in life and that's true in business as well. "People come into your life for a reason, a season or a lifetime." You have to understand that sometimes people come to you for certain needs and once those needs are meet, they must move on so that they can continue their own journey into discovery. We as hairdressers have an extreme power over people, which is why they are drawn to us. What we do for them behind the chair is a huge part of their self-esteem, and sometimes they need more than what we can provide so they search elsewhere to get their life needs met.

One of the hardest things to accept is that they've chosen not to seek your services any longer (for whatever reason). Don't feel too badly - sometimes they come back, sometimes they don't. You just have to understand that your purpose with that client has been fulfilled, and you will be ready to begin a new relationship with the next client that comes through the door. Isn't that the beauty of our business with people?

Open Your Eyes

Having clients not return to you is also a great way for you to evaluate yourself and perhaps the way you conduct your business. It gives you an eye opener to help you to stay focused and humble. You realize that you can't take anyone for granted, and must VALUE each and every client that you get the opportunity to service. Clients have many options down the street, and it is up to you to maintain a positive feeling to entice that client to continue to return to you!

Check yourself and think about the last few visits you had with the clients that did not return.

- Did you do all your homework?

- Did you give them the BEST of you?

- Did you offer something new if it was a long time client?

- Were you in the mood?

Unfortunately, clients know when we are not "ON" and that has a huge impact on they way they perceive their experience with us.

Fake It

As a hairdresser, "the show must go on" no matter how we feel. We have to learn how to "fake it till you make it" because clients depend on our personalities to help them feel good. You have to smile even if you feel like crying and when you're not in the mood, you need to dig deep down inside and pull it out of yourself. It builds fantastic character in us, so everyone is a winner!

Learn The Lesson

People come into our lives to teach us something about ourselves that we may not have yet discovered. Our purpose is to unravel the best in them and in return we discover the best in ourselves. It is such a beautiful business; developing relationships with people from all walks of life. There are many life lessons we learn on a daily basis if we only take the time to see what it is that we can see through each other and what it is that we truly offer as human beings. Every day that we encounter another soul in our chair is another piece of life yet to reveal. Grow with your clients, learn from them, and embrace their presence in your chair and in your life!

Here are some ideas to re-connect with your clients:

- Don't throw out old client information – you never know when they may return!
- Send out a periodic newsletter via postal mail or email or post it to your web site.
- Offer punch cards for services and retail (once they use up a certain number of punches or a specified dollar value, they receive a service/product at a discount or free).
- Host an "invitation-only" VIP event.

"A big shot is just a little shot who keeps on shooting."
Ray Baker

Tips & Snips

Three things I will do to regain my lost clients:

1. _____

2. _____

3. _____

COME ONE, COME ALL, TO THE GREATEST SHOW OF ALL!

Are you ready to be inspired? Do you value your profession enough to want to explore the many possibilities within your career? Do you want to get excited all over again about being in this fantastic industry? Then be a participator and come to the shows!

It's Worth The Money

Going to Beauty Trade shows is worth more than the investment of time and money. The long time benefits you receive from the short time that you are there well exceeds your expectations, IF you attend with the right mindset. If the main reason you are going is just because you need continuing hours and you have no real interest in learning anything new, then surely, your time will be wasted. But, if you go to the show with the intent of connecting to your profession and looking for opportunities to reevaluate what you already know, then you come back to the salon inspired again, and your time spent was successful. Beauty Shows are designed to encourage salon professionals to challenge themselves to the next level of their career. They offer an exchange of ideas from one professional to another in all areas of this business. That alone is worth the trip.

Take Advantage Of The Show

Before you go to a show, you should create a plan of action. Don't walk around without having a purpose. Before the show you should review the companies who will be there and jot down which ones you are interested in seeing. All manufacturers are trying to get you to come to their booth, so select your first choices then go where the excitement draws you. You will always be distracted from your action plan because there is so much going on. But if you keep to your focus, then you will be satisfied with your time invested. There is an enormous amount of action at shows, so you have to decide what will be of benefit to your needs as a professional.

Leaders And Mentors

Everyone needs education. You cannot grow in this business without learning and refreshing all facets of being a beauty professional. Manufacturers take pride in developing top-notch educators and leaders to educate you in areas that will be of benefit to your future. Finding a leader that you can relate to will encourage you to sharpen up your skills whether they would be in technical areas or in business. Mentors are your link to the future and a mark to the past. They help you by readying you to move forward and be a bigger part of our industry. They motivate and encourage you to look beyond what you do everyday behind the chair, and see the profession in a new light.

Network, Network, Network

Besides all the new products, new tools, new techniques, new outlook you receive from attending the beauty trade shows, one of the most rewarding and fulfilling reasons to come is all the people you meet. Think about it, everyone there is a beauty professional, and where you have beauty professionals you have conversation. Our industry is filled with chatty individuals; we love to share our insight and ideas with each other. It's our way of expressing our passion for this industry. Talking with other professionals offers different points of view on topics that may be affecting you or your salon, or perhaps they share a new career direction they are venturing into, or a business idea that you didn't know about. Socializing at the show is the greatest parting gift you will receive from attending. The networking possibilities are endless, and the bonding experience can be just what you and your salon needed.

Learn! Move on! Grow! Go to the Show!

50 WAYS TO TREAT YOUR CLIENT

Service is everything…

Did you ever walk into a salon where you felt like you were being a bother more than they actually wanted your patronage? Or even worse, a snooty clerk told you to "sign in and take a seat". What kind of business-building is that? No warm welcome hello, no "someone will be right with you", or even an acknowledgment of what service you would like to have done.

This lack of business ethics happens in our industry and it is a shame those salons are even patronized!

Treating your clients right is a big part of your position as a beauty professional.

Our profession is about making clients feel good as well as look good, and it is in our best interest to treat our clients with the respect and appreciation they deserve for choosing our salon for their services.

Remember…It is in the whole experience that a client determines his or her judgment on whether he or she will return.

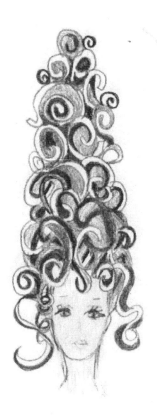

50 WAYS TO" TREAT" YOUR CLIENT

1. Give them a warm welcome

2. Offer refreshing beverage in a nice glass

3. Choose appropriate music

4. Burn aromatherapy

5. Smile

6. Listen more than talk

7. Ask a lot of questions regarding their lifestyle and beauty concerns

8. Give a shampoo, facial, or other treatments they'll remember

9. Keep your station clean

10. Brush off their neck and face after a cutting service to keep them clean

11. Explain what you're doing when you see them watching you

12. Demonstrate your products to show them how they work

13. Teach your clients what to do

14. Clean up their face during a color application

15. Offer current magazines

16. Make suggestions for something new

17. Hold special events

18. Send birthday cards

19. Offer monthly specials

20. Write a newsletter with news of your salon, upcoming events, beauty tips, and product/service updates. Mail to your clients or post on your web site.

21. Do free services for a client in need

22. Send a sick client a get well card

23. Take an older client to the movies

24. Be nice, always

25. Thank clients for coming in

26. Give away a hug. Be a happy hugger

27. Take your client even though she is late

28. Talk to them, look in their eyes

29. Enjoy giving the service, it shows

30. Be kind to fellow workers, clients are watching

31. Bring in new services, products, and people

32. Offer tips of the trade on health and beauty

33. Acknowledge "life events" (baby, wedding, graduation)

34. Introduce clients to each other

35. Hold a client contest; it's fun!

36. Make a house call if necessary

37. Throw a client-appreciation party

38. Network with clients' businesses; hold an open house for all clients with small business

39. Hold a benefit for a client or family member in need

40. Suggest fun and educational web-sites and books

41. Be organized

42. Be professional

43. Educate yourself. Go to hair or beauty events

44. Dress for success

45. Keep yourself healthy, exercise, eat right, think positive

46. "BE THERE" in the moment of the service

47. Show appreciation for their continued support

48. Be cheerful

49. Accommodate Accommodate, Accommodate

50. Be proud of your profession

Real success is when a client leaves with a smile and returns with a friend.

"Do the best you know how, and that's it."
Bob Provenzano (my "Pops")

Tips & Snips

Write three nice things you will do today for your clients:

1. _____

2. _____

3. _____

ENDLESS OPPORTUNITIES IN BUSINESS

Brilliant business begins with understanding your opportunities! The concept of a fantastic business is not only about the bottom line, but also how your work fulfills you and how you affect other people along the road. There is a business code to always remember and to continue to pass along as you grow in this business. That code is "OPO", which stands for Other People Oriented. Make sure that your main concern is other people and not yourself first. Such a simple concept, yet so overlooked. It is the way to begin your business with a commitment to integrity and to develop people skills that will take you all the way to the bank. Incorporating the understanding of people and their emotions will provide for your continual growth in your career and your business, no matter which avenue of the industry you choose.

Don't Limit Yourself

Don't limit yourself to one aspect of business. There is a whole world of possibilities within our industry that will allow you to embrace passions besides the option of being a hairdresser. You have to be able to stay open-minded. Don't become what everyone else is. Be your own star right where you are or be a star where *you* want to go.

Discovering uniqueness in your career evolves in the process of personal growth, as well as within the journey of your career. Opportunities seem to arise when you are mentally ready to move on and can sense a strong desire for something more. My uniqueness has shown up at different stages of my life. I discovered that I had talent in a diverse range of areas simply by the experiences I encountered.

When I first began, I found my talent in cutting. Over time, my strength became makeovers. I then expressed myself through competing and photo work. Next, I found gratification in teaching. Now I find passion through my writing. I believe that you discover your personal uniqueness as your life unfolds.

Discover your own uniqueness. Whether it is: that you like numbers, or you have a creative flair, that you like photo work or education, or enjoy sales - the point is that there are plenty of opportunities for you to learn as you grow within the business.

Always remember that there is plenty of room at the top.

Stop, Look, And Listen

You have to stop and take a good look around you to see your opportunities and find out more about the arena that you're interested in. Find a mentor and study their work to find out how they got where you want to go. Then, ask if there is any way that you can assist them or observe them, even if it is for free. Trade magazines offer a great source for information. They focus on all aspects of the industry and they tell you where you can find what you're looking for. Check the table of contents or in the back for resources.

Life Skills

You have a wealth of information about every subject, every business, every day. Your most valuable resource is your clients. They can provide education that some people go to school for years to understand. It is all in the way we value it. If you listen more, you'll be surprised to see how much information we have access to. We have our own network of people right in front of us that can and would be willing to offer us information on anything we ask about. Why? Because we have built a *relationship* with them, a connection that keeps our business growing.

Challenge Yourself

Take one full day of taking notes after each client - find out about their jobs, what hobbies they have, who they invest with, who cleans for them, etc. You'll be surprised to see all the diverse subjects we talk about and how they can benefit you or someone that you know. It is so *amazing* what we are exposed to every day. Sometimes we forget that the whole world is in our hands! So pay attention!

Key To Success

Your approach is the key to your success. It is HOW you deal with people that will affect the way your business is viewed. People come back to you for the way you make them feel - in the beauty business, or in any other business. Think about it. Why do you keep returning to your favorite business? Usually, it's because of that one person with whom you did business. It is the way he or she made you feel. The return rate of customers is primarily based on positive human experiences. It is an exchange of emotions as well as technical aptitude and a comfortable atmosphere that brings a customer back. Business is just business without being OPO (Other People Oriented) first. Successful businesses know OPO and place value in knowing that *is* their business.

Image

Create your own IMAGE, your own STYLE of doing business, and your OWN relationships with the people you need to know. Ask if you don't know the answer. Pick up the phone to do your homework with things you don't understand. No one will think less of you. People love to share their knowledge. There is an information highway all around us that we can forever learn and grow from. This is the era of "all for one and one for all". Be a cheerleader for everyone around you and you will be pleasantly surprise at just how much enthusiasm and cooperation you will receive!

Walk the Walk. Talk the Talk. That is BUSINESS!

"Learn from all than you know."
Unknown

Tips & Snips

What will you do today to remember to pay attention to what is in front of you?

1. _____

2. _____

3. _____

PLANNING FOR SUCCESS

Want to be successful in life and in business? Follow what highly successful people and companies have in common:

A PLAN

1. Put your goals in writing:

   There is a remarkable difference between saying what you desire to do and putting it in writing.

   Example: This week's goal is to make $xxx, sell xxx product and find xxx new clients.

2. Be specific:

   Focus on what you can accomplish, not what you can't. State your intentions clearly.

   Example: I will up-sell my existing clients to more services and pass out 3 business cards per day.

3. Make it measurable:

Set a date for a deadline.

Example: By the end of the month I will have <u>xxx</u> new clients, sold $<u>xxx</u> in retail, <u>xxx</u> new color services, and <u>xxx</u> perms.

> *"Unfortunately, the dollar dictates what we can and cannot have. But what it does not determine is the quality of the human spirit inside of us."*
>
> *Patti Misunis*

Tips & Snips

Write down your goals for your career:

_____

_____

_____

_____

_____

_____

THE CONNECTION

Did you ever stop to think of why a client returns to a salon year after year? Is it the warm welcome from the receptionist at the front desk? The all-new check-your-e-mail-while-you-process at the café? Or is it the mini neck massage you received at the shampoo bowl? Granted, these are all fantastic amenities to incorporate into your salon's marketing efforts, targeting new clients as well as keeping your existing ones excited. But what really brings back the client year after year is the one-on-one human touch connection between the client and the stylist; the relationship that transpires out of trust and personal experience.

I honor the fact that the "latest" trends in services and products are a great way to lure the client in the salon doors, but the fact is, what truly makes a client return year after year, decade after decade is the connection you have built between yourself and your client; that very human and irreplaceable factor that makes or breaks the experience the client has. Clients come to us for so much more than our expertise - they come to receive validation for who they are and where they are in their life. The most important skill they never taught you in beauty school was how to deal with the many different personalities you come into contact with daily.

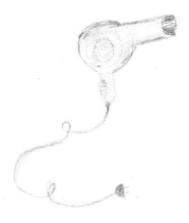

When a client comes to you, he or she has a story to tell and usually it is about what is happening in his or her life. Their hair is a huge reflection on what is going on. You have the golden tools to make that client not only look good, but you also have the ability to make them feel magnificent. What happens in your chair has a big impact on another human being. They look to you as a role model with all the necessary goods to "fix" them and their self-image. Wow! What a thought! Your work, on their head, plays a significant part in their life's events.

Think about it. How many times have you had to comfort your client through your hair session to help her or him feel better about what was going on in their life? Clients come to us because they place value in what we have to offer them spiritually. We add a rainbow of color to people's lives that few else can provide. This, I believe, is the gift that we have to offer: our personal touch that comes from our heart to theirs. This service cannot be bought, nor can it be eliminated. It is the sunshine that you provide to another human being - the connection is what they treasure. The time you spend with them personally. As time flies by and the years go on, you might wonder why you are still standing behind that chair, and then you'll reflect back at all the lives you have touched and the ones that have touched yours and you will remember. Be proud to be a hairdresser!

"The language of love is understood by all."

Unknown

Tips & Snips

Reflect at the end of your day...your true treasure(s):

_____

_____

_____

_____

_____

EPILOGUE

This book has allowed me to share my down-to-earth approach to help you get to where you want to be in this industry. My common sense insights are for anyone who desires positive energy injected into their career. You have just experienced my selection of strategies that I firmly believe will effectively build your enthusiasm for your personal success.

Happiness to all...

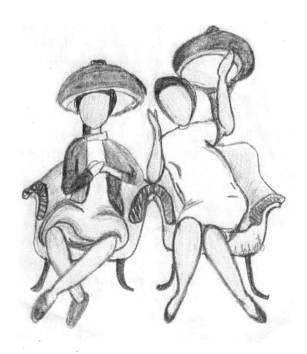

ABOUT THE AUTHOR

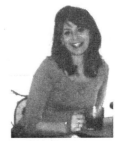

Kathy Jager is a twenty-five year veteran in cosmetology, living in a Chicago suburb with her husband, Marty, and two daughters, Camille and Marie. Kathy has a diverse background in cosmetology, education, and business. She is a vivacious, creative self-starter who strives to remain current in the industry's progressive path by challenging herself to enrich her life and business and add new horizons to her journey. Her passion for her work and the inner and outer beauty of her clients is contagious. Her infectious personality and enthusiasm for life has everyone leaving her salon with a smile.

In *As The Chair Turns…Tips and Snips of Advice for Your Journey Behind the Chair*, Kathy shares with her peers the passion, knowledge and experiences of her successful career. Nothing gets her more excited than to be able to help people reach their desired dreams!

Kathy Jager is now offering an inspirational and educational seminar focused on designing and developing your personal success.

The author welcomes your comments, and can be reached at:

Kathy Jager
15110 LaPorte
Oak Forest, IL 60452
Email: mkj151@aol.com

Additional copies of this book may be purchased at:
http://www.lulu.com/pros-grapevine